A Comprehensive Guide to the Fundamentals of Travel Nursing

For the Beginning or Aspiring
Professional

A Comprehensive Guide to the Fundamentals of Travel Nursing:

For the Beginning or Aspiring Professional

by Emma Pointer

ISBN-13: 9781704736075

This material has been prepared for informational purposes only, and is not intended to provide, and should not be relied on for, tax, legal or accounting advice. You should consult your own tax, legal and accounting advisors.

Table of Contents

INTRODUCTION   IV

WHAT IS TRAVEL NURSING AND IS IT FOR ME?   1

How much nursing experience do I need to be a travel nurse?   4
Why do hospitals need travel nurses?   8
How does travel nursing pay work?   10
What are duplicated expenses?   18
Where will I live when travel nursing?   24
Can I bring my pets or a travel partner?   27
Where can I go and how does licensing work?   31
Do I get benefits as a travel nurse?   34

REVIEW WHAT YOU HAVE LEARNED SO FAR   36

ACTION PLAN   42

Outline Your "Why"   44
Speak with Family and Friends   49
Downsize and Minimize   52
Finances   55
Getting a Recruiter and an Agency   61
Build Your Profile   69
Get Your License   72
Plan for Your Permanent Job   75
Talk to Co-Workers You Trust   77
Submit to a Job   80
Interview   83
Accept an Offer   86
Complete Onboarding   91
Secure Housing   93
Pack and GO!   95

BONUS CONTENT   98

Introduction

Bill rates, hourly rates, taxed income, untaxed stipends, duplicating expenses, contract negotiation, working with recruiters, securing housing, compact and non-compact licenses, insurance and benefits, profiles, job submissions, onboarding... It's all like an entirely new world that can no doubt be incredibly intimidating at first and difficult to navigate. The purpose of this book is to not let those possibly new ideas and topics deter you from or slow you down in your journey to reaching your goal of becoming a travel nurse.

Although these topics can be boring and dry, this book takes you step-by-step in a casual tone as if you are learning these things from a friend. While much of this information can be found online, the format here is unique as it is presented as a guide to your journey that will not be your only source of information but rather your foundation to help keep your research quick and on track.

Throughout this guide, you are encouraged to question the material presented and apply it to your specific situation and seek out more information as needed. This way, you aren't flipping through a bunch of pages that go on and on about things that don't apply to you. For example, the option of travel nursing in an RV is presented in this guide. If that is going to be your thing, please get much more information on that than is presented in this book before you do it. The internet is powerful. A simple search "travel nursing in an RV" will provide you with weeks worth of reading. However, most of us aren't interested in living in an RV and don't want to pay for information on it. The reason this guide is so unique is that without it presented here, you may never think to do the search "travel nursing in an RV" because you may not even know it's an option. With just independent internet research, you may be missing out on important steps and opportunities that could perfectly fit your needs. The goal here is to give you a complete overview of your options and the basic knowledge you need to explore those options fully. While we do go over facts and basic knowledge, the focus here is more on the process.

The following guide is divided into two sections. The first section "What is travel nursing and is it for me?" challenges you to look at the role of the travel nurse and the obstacles it presents while applying it to your own life. In addition to highlighting potential obstacles, the first section also helps you understand the basics of travel nursing.

In the second section, "Action Plan", you are guided step-by-step in the creation of an actionable plan that concludes with the first day of your first travel assignment. This action plan teaches along the way about common misunderstandings for each step and various approaches for each task. Upon completion of this book and the steps outlined within it, you can expect to be fully prepared to land a job as a travel nurse and start your first travel nursing assignment with confidence.

As a travel nurse myself, I know exactly how much this change in your life means to you and I'm here to help you navigate it as smoothly as possible. When I started, I did the research without a guide and it took me months and I ran into a lot of dead ends. Fueled by my passion for teaching (my Master's degree is in Nursing Education), all the knowledge I have gathered through my own experience, and the hole I found when I was doing the same thing that you are about to, I decided to put this together for others to use. I'm so excited for you to get started and to be your guide at the beginning of this amazing journey that is going to lead you to more financial freedom, diverse experience to further your career, and adventures to remember for a lifetime. Feel free to reach out to me directly on my TTTNursing social media platforms if you run into any issues!

As a bonus, this is your official invitation to join the exclusive TTTNursing Facebook group for personalized feedback and follow up on the material covered in this book with me and other aspiring travel nurses like you (Travel Nursing for Beginners- TTTNursing). Additionally, I have put out several informational videos on my TTTNursing YouTube channel about travel nursing as well.

What is travel nursing and is it for me?

So, you have probably heard a little about travel nursing, maybe your cousin has a friend who did it and loves it. It is possible you know more than a little. Regardless, let's take a minute to go right back to the basics. In this section, we are going to touch on the fundamentals that everyone considering travel nursing should have a full understanding of.

Leaving the stability of your permanent job and the security of the city you know so well is nothing to take lightly. As you read through this section, try to put the glamorous images that your cousin's friend is CONSTANTLY posting on social media of her place on contract in Hawaii out of your head. Instead, really think about what this would mean for your life, goals, and well-being.

Travel nursing is a life-changing adventure but it truly is NOT a good lifestyle for everyone. There is nothing wrong with that. Travel nursing is not all that it is portrayed to be on social media and in the blog posts.

In this section, we will try to get a realistic understanding of what it means to be a travel nurse. It is better to realize the truth now rather than when you are stuck crying, alone in a hotel in North Dakota on your days off when you expected to be relaxing on the beach in Florida.

We will go through all the common questions that people have about travel nursing with an un-sugarcoated, simple approach to make sure this choice is right for you. Feel free to take notes as you go and re-read sections until you have a full understanding.

This stuff can be overwhelming and confusing but don't get discouraged. Take it one section at a time and feel free to write down additional questions to do extra research on. These topics are HUGE and many people spend months researching before they decide to take the jump. Use these prompts as a starting point to learn what you don't know or a refresher on what you have learned so far before you continue and create your action plan.

How much nursing experience do I need to be a travel nurse?

We are going to start out heavy here. This is possibly the MOST asked question with the most dreaded response because people are excited to get started. But, good things come to those who wait!

Short answer: Two years of experience in the specialty you plan to travel in is most often recommended and required.

That being said, if you do not have at least two years don't close the book and stop reading just yet. To be in a place where you are fully ready to be a travel nurse, (keep reading to find out how to get there) takes a lot of preparing and planning. If you aren't at the two-year mark yet, you may be there before you even feel ready. Additionally, this, like most other things in life, is just a recommendation. There are recruiters who will try to place you with a year of experience and hospitals that will hire you. Keep in mind that it is your nursing license on the line. Thus, it is your responsibility to be real with yourself about when you are ready.

No matter the amount of experience you have there are several important points to note here. The minute you decide you are eventually going to be a travel nurse, start preparing at work. This may mean different things for different people.

The first suggestion is to **become comfortable with being uncomfortable**. Volunteer to float to a different unit, see if there are any openings in the resource pool at your hospital, get a PRN job at a different hospital in your city. Try going outside your comfort zone (your home unit at your home hospital) and see how you feel. If without the security of your co-workers and familiar environment, you feel overwhelmed, you may want to get some more experience before jumping into travel nursing.

The second suggestion is to **make sure you love your specialty**. The best time to switch specialties is at your permanent job. Once you start traveling, the hospitals are not going to hire you on a labor and delivery floor if you are a med surg nurse. If your dream is to go into critical care try to make the switch now, put in your two years and then you will be able to travel within the specialty that you love. Also, keep in mind that some specialties pay better than others depending on supply and demand. Making a switch might be worth it in the long run but once you start traveling you can always take a break and go back to permanent staff to make a specialty transition.

We should also quickly touch on experience with charting systems. As nurses, a large part of what we do is chart we what did. We also rely on charting systems to help us find information about our patients quickly and keep us on track with giving meds and other tasks. How many charting systems do you have experience with? How much do you rely on the charting system to make you feel comfortable? How would you react if your hospital decided to change systems? These are important questions to ask yourself because many different charting systems are used throughout the US. As a travel nurse, you may expect to not know where to find a toothbrush for your patient but you may be surprised to also not know how to find their lab values in the chart if you are unfamiliar with the system. Flexibility and comfortability asking for help are key. It also doesn't hurt to have experience using several different charting systems.

Why do hospitals need travel nurses?

Obviously, I know, because they don't have enough staff nurses to take care of all the patients they have. But this should be relevant to your decision to become a travel nurse. Why don't they have enough staff nurses? For some places, maybe you are covering maternity leaves, filling the gap during the increased census for flu season, or holding down the fort until they can get a new hire trained because someone just retired. For other places, the reasons might not be as reassuring. Perhaps the management is poor and everyone who works there gets burnt out and leaves. Maybe the hospital is poorly run and the environment is off-putting to nurses.

Whatever the reason, as a travel nurse you have to expect to walk into a storm of a hospital. They need you for a reason. Staffing and moral is probably bad. If that is not the case, wonderful. But just realize, they are paying a premium to have you there, and there is some reason they are willing to pay that.

This connects back to the previous question regarding experience. Knowing that the hospital that you walk into may not be the ideal work environment, your experience becomes that much more important. When everything is going wrong, you will want your experience as a levelheaded well-prepared nurse to lean on. At the end of the day, you need to know how to help your patients and what to document to prove you did. Nursing is essentially the same no matter where you go or who you are with. Have a great knowledge base, positive attitude, and patient-centered mindset and you will be able to handle whatever the world of healthcare throws your way.

How does travel nursing pay work?

One of the HUGE perks of travel nursing is the pay. It also can be confusing at first but it shouldn't be! Let's go through the basics so you can make the decision if this would be something that might work for your unique financial situation.

A couple of basic terms regarding travel nurse pay that you should be aware of:

Taxable income: Taxable income is what gets reported to the IRS as your wages. The amount of taxes you pay is also determined by and withdrawn from your taxable income. Additionally, if you go to rent an apartment, get a new loan or line of credit, or anything else that requires you to disclose how much money you make, this will be the amount that you report.

Untaxable income: In the world of travel nursing pay packages, untaxable income is money that your agency allots to you to cover your living and travel expenses, including housing and meals. This money does not get taxes taken out from it and is not reported in your yearly income since it is essentially repayment for the money you are spending to be able to do your job. This stipend is only available to you if you are duplicating expenses (we will cover this in the next section). The maximum amount that the agency is able to pay you in this category is set by the government (The General Services Administration commonly known as the GSA) depending on the location that you are working in and the cost of living there. You can find the most recent GSA travel per diem rates by doing a search online and entering the zip code of the city you are planning on working in on the GSA website. Agencies are not always able to pay travelers the maximum allowed GSA rate. It depends on what bill rate is for the job.

When a recruiter sends you a pay package, realize that these numbers are usually flexible and negotiable depending on your circumstances. There may be some room to get a higher taxable wage and a lower stipend depending on the agency. It is best to consult a tax advisor who has experience working with untaxable travel stipends to see what you will be looking for in a pay package.

Also, keep in mind that most travel nurses will opt to find their own housing on contract and get paid a housing stipend. However, it may be possible to find an agency that provides housing. In that case, you should not be receiving any untaxable stipends for housing. If the agency provides housing, you may still get untaxed stipends to cover meals.

Bill rate: The bill rate is what the agency bills the hospital per hour for the nurse's work. This is usually much more than what the nurse actually receives on their paycheck from their agency per week since the agency needs to take money from this as well to be able to pay its bills.

Hourly rate: What the nurse is getting paid by the agency per hour for their work. This is the offer that the nurse receives from the agency after the agency subtracts the money they need to pay their bills.

Travel nurses are usually paid weekly by their travel agencies. The travel agency is in charge of taking the bill rate and dividing it out to cover their expenses and then pay the nurse. It is the agency that decides what percentage of the bill rate the nurse receives. This is how pay can vary between agencies for the same job at the same hospital. One agency may have more expenses to run their company and thus not be able to pay the nurse as much as a different agency that has fewer expenses.

Bill rates are not typically advertised to nurses. The amount that is taken out goes to many different places and people thus sometimes making the bill rate MUCH different than the nurse's hourly rate. There is no set percentage of a bill rate that the nurse should receive.

The bill rate goes to fund everything that the agency does. This is important to remember when comparing agencies. Any perk that you are getting from the agency is being paid for out of the bill rate. So, more perks usually mean less money in your pocket. For this reason, it may be wise to not pay attention to all the "wonderful" benefits that a recruiter presents that are provided by their agency.

The more "free" benefits being offered, the less of the bill rate left over for your paycheck. Some agencies will send nurses flowers on the first day of their assignment or gift cards to congratulate them for landing a contract. Some people may appreciate the thought from the agency. Some may rather work with an agency that keeps things simple and instead of flowers adds an extra $40 divided out into their hourly rate over the contract. The point is that the bill rate is set in stone but there are many ways that it can get divided depending on the agency.

Here is an example of a pay package that may be presented (actual dollar amounts of the offer will depend on the specialty and location of the contract):

EXAMPLE PAY PACKAGE	
ASSIGNMENT	(SPECIALTY) RN IN (LOCATION)
DATES	(MAY LIST ONE START DATE HERE OR MAY LIST SEVERAL FLEXIBLE DATES)
DETAILS	36 HOURS/WEEK FOR 13 WEEKS
WEEKLY GROSS	$1,800, COMBINED HOURLY RATE : $50
PAY BREAKDOWN	(TAXED HOURLY: $20, UNTAXED HOURLY: $30, TRAVEL ALLOWANCE: $500

In this example, we see that $1,800 a week is the offer. However, of that $1,800, only $720 a week ($20 an hour for 36 hours) will be taxed. The nurse who accepts this offer can expect $1,080 a week tax-free to use on housing and meals and $720 minus tax for taxable income.

Additionally, in this offer, the agency is providing a $500 travel bonus. How this is paid will depend on the agency. Some agencies give a $250 bonus at the beginning of the assignment for travel expenses and a $250 bonus at the end to travel home. Other agencies give all $500 at the beginning. It may even be possible to negotiate to have the $500 added into your hourly rate and spread out over the contract if that would be beneficial to you.

Whether or not the bonus is taxed also depends on the agency and how they structure the payout. If it is a travel allowance, it really shouldn't be taxed since it is a reimbursement for money that you spent to get to the contract. However, some agencies will classify a similar amount of money as a completion bonus, thus taxing it at the flat rate set by the federal government for taxing bonuses.

What are duplicated expenses?

Duplicated expenses are a tax-related issue. As with any tax-related issue, it is best to find a tax agent that specializes in travel taxes to discuss your unique circumstances and any recent changes to the tax laws. The following advice is meant for the beginner and may not apply to your situation.

As discussed in the previous section, travel nursing may make how you deal with your taxes much different since most people are not used to handling the complications that come with receiving tax-free stipends and per diem pay. When a bit of time is set aside to grasp the basic principles and stipulations per diem payments, expensive mistakes are avoided and the whole idea seems much less daunting. If you are confused by the jargon, consider looking to a professional for advice or following the basic requirements outlined here.

Travel tax is complex and could make up an entire book itself if we were to go through all the options so instead, we will cover the most common and simplest option which is to duplicate expenses and spend time at you tax home. If, after reading this section, you decide this option is not ideal for you, some starting places for more research may be looking into being an "itinerant employee" or the option of maintain a job at your tax home instead of maintaining a residence (may not be as simple as it sounds and usually is not recommended but may be worth looking into).

The simplest and most common way to get the stipends tax-free is to duplicate expenses and to spend time at your tax home.

Duplicating expenses is maintaining a residence in your home state AND paying for a place to stay 7 days a week wherever your contract is.

Spending time at your tax home is achieved by maintaining finances near your tax home (keep your bank address as your permanent address/tax home) and ties there (return home and spend a recommended 30 days out of the year there).

Note that for your residence in your home state, you have the option of owning a house and paying for upkeep and property taxes, having a mortgage, or paying fair market value rent.

Note that for your duplication residence (the place you are staying close to your contract), if you only pay for a hotel room the 3 nights of the week you work, you will not be able to get the full stipend untaxed. Since it is a daily allotted amount, you may get the stipend for 3 out the 7 days. For example, if the stipend quoted by the recruiter is $1,000 for housing and meals per week, that would be equivalent to $143 per day. So, if you are duplicating expenses for 3 out of the 7 days you may only be eligible to receive $429 out of the $1,000. As long as you make your agency aware of this they may be able to adjust the amount of untaxed stipends you are receiving and increase your taxed hourly rate. If you wrongfully receive tax-free stipends and get audited you will have to pay back taxes and fines.

You may choose an option that does not include duplicating expenses but if that is the case you should talk with a tax advisor and your agency. You may need to let your agency know you will need your whole pay package to be taxable wages. Some people will go this route when they take an assignment close to home and do not need to find living arrangements because they are able to return home each night. Be aware that if your agency presents you with a pay package that is entirely taxable income the gross amount will likely be less than the gross amount of the package with tax-free stipends. This is because the agency has to account for the increase in payroll taxes that they will be paying by presenting the pay package as entirely taxable.

Be aware that if audited you must be able to prove you were duplicating expenses. So, don't pay your mom fair market value rent for a room in her house using cash. Pay rent with checks so you have a record. Look at listings in your area for comparable living arrangements and print some off to keep with your tax records in case you need to prove fair market value.

If you own your home or pay a mortgage, be careful with renting it out while you are gone. If you plan on renting out your place for an extended lease (12 months or more), you need to reserve at least one room in the house for yourself that isn't occupied by a renter. That way you are able to return home and stay in that room throughout the year. Conversely, you may also choose to rent it out short term (less than the full 12 months of the year) and have it available and empty for you to stay in when you return home.

As mentioned, this tax stuff can get complicated. Before taking the jump into travel nursing consult your trusted travel tax agent to make sure you have all your boxes checked and there are no surprises at tax time.

Where will I live when travel nursing?

Some people are creative with living arrangements when travel nursing. There are three basic options: furnished, mobile or unfurnished.

The first is the most common. Most people will find **a furnished place to stay** near the hospital they are working at. Many people offer furnished mother-in-law suites or finished basements equipped with kitchens for short term rental. You may also opt to stay in a furnished room in someone's home and share the common living area. Some travel nurses will travel with a group of one or two other nurses and share a furnished home. Also, an extended stay hotel is usually available in most cities but can be costly. Having a furnished place to stay is nice since most nurses drive to their assignments and only bring what fits in their car.

The second option would be to invest in **mobile living arrangements**. Some people have an RV that they move from assignment to assignment. They duplicate expenses by paying rent for space at an RV park. Other people have smaller mobile living arrangements like a converted van or trailer that they pay to park somewhere. This is a good option if you are looking to travel long term or already have the mobile living arrangement. However, if you are not sure if travel nursing is something you will be doing long term, the initial investment for an RV and truck may not be worth it. Mobile living arrangements help alleviate the struggle of packing up all your belongings and moving every 13 weeks but it may not be the best option for everyone.

The third and least common option is finding **unfurnished living arrangements**. This option can be expensive but some people make it work when they know they want to stay in an area for more than 13 weeks or are unable to find accommodations in the other two categories. This requires you to buy or bring the basic necessities like a bed and kitchenware. Many people find things for sale second hand or cheap online. If you are comfortable living with the bare minimum and able to find an apartment complex that offers a short-term lease this could be beneficial. It also can be very costly if you aren't careful about it.

Wherever you decide to live on assignment, life will be a little different than it was back home. But, it can be freeing to live simply and have very little material possessions to hold you down. Trying out many different living arrangements can help you learn a lot about your wants and needs long term.

Can I bring my pets or a travel partner?

Absolutely! Many people travel with pets and partners. For pets, you may find that it can be a little more expensive and restricting for finding a place to live. Some renters have to pay pet fees and deposits and find that adds up quickly. Other renters have trouble finding housing that allows pets at all.

No matter the inconvenience, pets can be great to ease the loneliness of being away from home and everyone you know. It may make things harder or more expensive but you may find that it is very well worth it to you and it is definitely possible!

As far as partners/spouses/children, the more the merrier! Some families will all travel together and the spouse that isn't the nurse will home school the kids (there are many great resources online to help with this). Some families opt to take a single contract during the summer and treat it as an extended vacation!

For families, the most popular option tends to be mobile living arrangements as it can be especially difficult to find short term rentals with adequate private space. It is also difficult to pack up and move the amount of stuff that a whole family typically owns every 13 weeks. It certainly isn't impossible to explore other options but mobile living tends to be the most comfortable.

If you don't have children, your spouse or partner can absolutely travel with you as well. If you both are nurses get a recruiter who is willing to place a pair. Sometimes both of you can work at the same hospital. Other times a recruiter will opt to place you in hospitals within commuting distance from each other. If you are married or sharing finances be sure to do some research on tax restrictions regarding both of you taking full and untaxed housing stipends and sharing housing.

If the travel partner is not a nurse there are other options as well. Many couples find that the increase of income that comes with traveling is adequate for the spouse not to work and take care of the house and help with finding new assignments, housing, and planning fun stuff to do on days off.

Other travel partners find remote work or temporary jobs. See the list for a few ideas to get you started! Don't feel limited by this list. Be creative! It is easier than ever to find jobs making money online and also to advertise your services online and find customers!

Work for Traveling Partners

- HOMEMAKER
- REMOTE WORK WITHIN THEIR FIELD
- HANDYMAN
- MOW YARDS
- BLOG/WRITE ARTICLES ONLINE
- WORKING IN THE FOOD INDUSTRY
- BARTENDING
- RETAIL WORK (ESPECIALLY AROUND THE HOLIDAYS)
- DRIVING FOR RIDESHARE COMPANIES
- DRIVING FOR ON DEMAND FOOD DELIVERY COMPANIES
- DRIVING FOR ON DEMAND GROCERY DELIVERY COMPANIES
- DOG WALKING
- DOG SITTING
- TEMPORARY WORK THROUGH A TEMP AGENCY
- WORK AT RV PARK
- TRANSFER IN A JOB WITH LOCATIONS THROUGHOUT THE US
- START THEIR OWN BUSINESS (TRAVEL AGENT, PHOTOGRAPHER, CONSULTING, COACHING)
- BUY AND SELL ONLINE
- SOCIAL MEDIA MANAGEMENT
- AFFILIATE MARKETING
- COPYWRITING

#TTTNursing

Where can I go and how does licensing work?

You can be a travel nurse anywhere within the US (and some territories) that you are licensed in. Nursing licenses are either compact or non-compact depending on which state you are a permanent resident in. New legislation is always coming out regarding which states are compact so do an online search to see the most updated list.

If you have a compact license, you are able to travel to and work in any other compact state without getting and maintaining a license specifically for that state. Having residency in a compact state is ideal as licensing can get costly (although agencies frequently reimburse licensing costs if you secure a contract in that state with them).

Your recruiter will be able to direct you on licensing requirements and processes. However, you should find out if the state you reside in is a compact license state and you should also find out if the state you want to work in is a compact license state. Know that if you want to go to a non-compact state or you are a resident of non-compact state getting a license can take some time so plan accordingly.

On the subject of locations, it is important to bust the myth that travel nurses only go to Hawaii, Florida, Colorado, California, and other places that are fun and warm. You have control over where you go so if you have your heart set on Hawaii, go for it. Although, realize you might end up waiting for a contract that barely pays your bills. It is well known in the travel industry that some places "pay in sunshine" meaning they get by with not paying as well because people want to be there so they will take lower offers.

There is nothing wrong with taking contracts in places that you enjoy. It all comes back to your reason for traveling and your goals. While it might not be ideal weather, a contract in the middle of winter in Wisconsin might be good for the bank account and you could meet some really great people. The most important thing with travel nursing job security is to be open with location. Needs change constantly and you may not always be able to score a contract in your first pick location. However, a good recruiter will likely be able to find SOME job for you relatively easily if you are open with location.

Do I get benefits as a travel nurse?

Travel nursing does not carry the same benefits as a permanent staff job might. Agencies will offer insurance but you may find it is much more expensive than you were paying at your staff job. Many agencies have a waiting period for the insurance to become active (30 days from the contract start date for example). Your coverage may also lapse if you are to take time off between contracts. Additionally, if you switch agencies you will have to switch insurances. Switching agencies is very common as different agencies have different contracts in various cities. For all of these reasons, some travelers get their own private insurance or opt to carry insurance from their spouse.

Other benefits like PTO and paid sick days are rare but can be found depending on the agency. Just remember, that any PTO is ultimately paid for from the bill rate. For this reason, some travelers would rather not have PTO and just save the extra money they earn on contract to take time off between contracts. When traveling, don't forget that you will likely not be adding to a company retirement plan. You can, however, find your own retirement plan and contribute to it with each paycheck.

Traditional benefits can prove a hassle as a travel nurse. On a positive note, travel nursing arguably compensates for what it lacks in traditional benefits in more nontraditional benefits. As a travel nurse, you may not earn PTO but you gain the freedom to take as many days off between contracts as your financial situation allows. You are also spending your four days off a week in a new, exciting place with plenty of weekend and day trips waiting outside your door.

Review What You Have Learned So Far

We have covered a lot of ground. Let's take a minute to review what we have been over and apply it to your situation. It is important to look back on your notes and follow up with gathering any more information you need in order to answer these questions. We need to know exactly what we are getting into before we move on to our action plan. Once you have solid answers to these questions you know that you understand the basics of travel nursing.

1. When is your target start date?

_____

_____

_____

_____

2. How experienced will you be within your specialty by this date?

_____

_____

_____

_____

3. What specialty will you be traveling in?

_____

_____

_____

_____

4. Are you comfortable with learning a new charting system? How many charting systems do you have experience with?

_____

_____

_____

5.   What questions do you still have about travel nurse pay? Do you understand the difference between taxed and untaxed pay and the bill rate and your hourly rate?

_____

_____

_____

_____

6.   What is your plan for getting or not getting tax free stipends? How will you maintain a tax home or what is your alternative? Are you confident that your plan meets all tax requirements?

_____

_____

_____

_____

7. Where will you live while travel nursing? What is your ideal living arrangement while on contract?

_____

_____

_____

_____

8. Do you plan to travel with a pet or a partner? What challenges will this create? What benefits does this have?

_____

_____

_____

_____

9. Is your home state a compact license state? Is the state you want to work in a compact license state? What does this mean for you?

_____

_____

_____

_____

10. What other questions do you have that need answered before moving forward?

_____

_____

_____

_____

_____

_____

_____

_____

Some final questions to help decide if travel nursing is for you:

	Where do you see yourself in 5 years?	Where do you see yourself in 10 years?
Your Career		
Your Personal Life		
Your Financial Life		

How does travel nursing help you reach these goals?	

What barriers does travel nursing create to reaching your goals?	

Action Plan

So, you have come this far. You have read through all the topics so far in this book, completed the questions at the end of the last section, gotten most of your questions answered, and now you are ready to get serious! First, CONGRATULATIONS this is going to be an amazing ride. Second, slow down, there is still a lot more to learn.

In this section, we are going to create an action plan that is going to guide you all the way up to the first day of your first travel nursing assignment! I would recommend reading this whole section so you know what to expect and then coming back to each section as you go through the process. These sections are packed full of information and helpful tips. Remember, stay organized, and stay focused on your goals. Let's dive in!

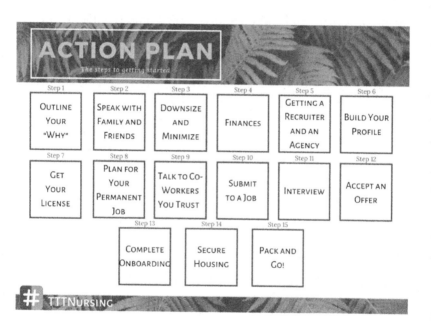

Outline Your "Why"

Speaking of staying organized and focused on your goals, the first step in this process is outlining and defining your goals. We touched on goals briefly in the previous section but we need to revisit the ideas now that we know the main goal involves travel nursing.

Every travel nurse has a unique life situation that puts them in the place to be able to travel. The unique situation determines where they get jobs, when they get jobs, and what they are looking for in a job. It is important to keep those reasons and goals at the front of your mind when thinking about anything travel nursing related and especially when making contract and housing decisions.

Before moving forward, I would encourage you to clearly define your goals. I am a visual person so I like to have my goals where I can see them every day. You can be crafty and make a sign to hang in your house, a wallpaper for your computer or phone or simply jot them down on a sticky note. I suggest using the following format:

WHY I am interested in travel nursing:

WHAT I am looking to gain from travel nursing:

WHAT I am willing to sacrifice to be a travel nurse:

WHAT I am most excited about:

Here is an example:

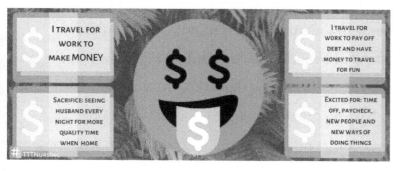

Put your creation somewhere you will see it often. It doesn't matter what your goals are as long as you stick to them. With the example presented above, this nurse would put a heavy focus on pay. From the goals outlined it seems they are traveling to better their finances. Perhaps traveling for them will mean less overtime and burn out than they had at their staff job. It may mean making all the money they need to make for the year in 6 months and then spending the rest of the time at home. It may mean working a bunch of overtime on contract then taking long breaks between contracts. Whatever it means, this nurse knows their goal is money. When looking at contracts and housing this nurse should keep money in the front of their mind. They shouldn't be distracted by location, day shift vs. night shift, agency perks or anything else that takes the attention from their goal. If your goal is money, go where the money is. A contract that does not fulfill your main goal will not make you happy.

An example on the opposite end would be if a nurse had the goal of being close to home. This nurse should be strictly focused and often remind themselves that being close to home is important to them. They shouldn't be distracted by money, other locations, or any other perks that would drive them away from their main goal; traveling close to home.

The examples are endless, but the main point is you have to pick what is most important to you and stick to it. There is a lot of pressure in the travel nursing world from recruiters who are trying to fill jobs. They will try to present you with options that may be nice but ultimately could give you a bad impression of travel nursing because they aren't right for you and your goals.

Know what you want and stick to it. Things that are less important to you, you may be willing to compromise on. Other things are make or break. Make a list now in your head that ranks the characteristics of a contract and their importance to you. Here are a few things that you may want to consider:

Most important

Least important

Location
Pay
Big city vs small town
Charting system
Hospital size
Trama level
If your preferred housing is available
Start date and end date
Day shift vs Night shift
Activities available on days off
Benefits (insurance, PTO)
Agency and agency policies

Speak with family and friends

Now that you are comfortable with the basic information associated with travel nursing and you have defined your "why" the next step is to share the exciting news with family and friends. I think this step is SO important for several reasons. First, it makes you accountable. You have decided this is something you are interested in, don't let the fear of the unknown hold you back. Tell people so that when you are still stuck at your staff job in 6 months, your Aunt Linda will ask you about travel nursing and you will be reminded that you are avoiding your dreams.

Second, the best way to learn is to teach. No matter how much you think you know, someone is always going to ask you a question that you may not know the answer to. At this point in your journey, you should be getting all your questions answered.

Discussing this adventure with a friend might bring up a topic or issue you hadn't thought to consider. Everyone looks at things differently, use it to your advantage.

Third, sometimes our friends and family know us better than we know ourselves. It might be good to talk the decision over with someone who has known you for a long time. They may be able to ground you and help you see things as they are, not how you want them to be. For example, if you discuss travel nursing with your longtime friend and explain that you are leaving to go across the country for 3 months and leaving the kids at home with their dad, he/she may be able to give you a reality check. They will remind you of the time you went Vegas with the girls for the weekend and came back to a house that was a disaster and kids who ate Pop-Tarts for breakfast, lunch, and dinner all weekend. Like with anything else, take advice from others with a grain of salt and always do what is best for you and your family. Perhaps your husband has become much more comfortable caring for a home and children since the Vegas trip and will do fine. Regardless, having outsider feedback can sometimes help big mistakes from being made.

You have to tell the people you love about your decision eventually. Do it early for these reasons. They may be sad to see you leave if they live nearby. But they will be happy for you when they see how excited you are about your new adventure. Plus, you can get them excited about planning a trip to come and see you wherever you end up!

Downsize and Minimize

Start to think about what you want to take with you when you travel. Downsizing and minimalizing apply to both your material possessions and your lifestyle. The biggest and most obvious area to downsize in is your material possessions. From the minute you decide to start travel nursing, before you buy anything think, "I am going to want to drag this from place to place with me every time I move?" This alone will make the whole process a lot easier. Stop bringing things you don't have space for into your life.

Also, start deciding what material possession are the most important to you. Can you live without a curling iron but need a hair straightener to function? Can you use a hair straightener to curl your hair? How about cooking? Do you really need a Crockpot, Instapot, Airfryer, blender, toaster oven, espresso maker, Keurig, griddle, AND a waffle maker? Decide which you can live without. Try it out for a week and see. All of this will make packing and deciding what to bring so much easier. A lot of times we don't even realize how little of the things we own we actually use.

Downsizing and minimalizing also apply to your life and lifestyle. Try to take time in the beginning stages to see if you are comfortable leaving behind certain parts of your life (like that on-again, off-again relationship that has been dragging you down). Practice giving things up that you know you will be sacrificing to travel and see how it makes you feel. This doesn't mean that you have to sit in your house and stare at the walls on your days off work. But, consider trying to go out to dinner by yourself instead of with your group of usual friends. Try to go to a social event where you don't know anyone. Or maybe you will be traveling in an RV with no cable TV, cut the cable now and explore your other options that are more mobile, like streaming shows online. If you slowly make these changes to your life it won't be so overwhelming when you actually leave and so many things change all at once.

Minimizing and downsizing for traveling doesn't mean deprivation or going without. It means being conscious of what is in your life and what kind of value it brings. When you limit what you have to only things you love and truly use and value, you become less overwhelmed by excess and have more time, energy, and space for what is important to you.

Finances

The next big step is to get your finances straight. While travel nursing can be financially lucrative, it can also be financially draining, especially at first. The costs upfront can be overwhelming and should be accounted for so you don't end up having to quit before you even start. To illustrate this fully we are going to look at a case study. I have seen the events that are laid out in this case study play out in real life MANY times to new travelers who are not prepared financially.

As you read through Bella's story, try to recognize the choices that she is making that are wrong. This is will be a good opportunity to review your knowledge and understanding of tax laws and finances associated with travel nursing. Learn from Bella's mistakes and put yourself in a position to not make the same ones.

Bella is a critical care nurse in South Carolina. She has three years of experience in med surg and a year and a half experience in a critical care unit at a level 3 trauma center. She is so excited about travel nursing, she used to work with a girl who did it and loves it. That ex-coworker gave her the name of their recruiter and within a couple of weeks, that recruiter had a job lined up for her in Seattle, WA. Bella did a little research online but got bored with it and just decided to go for it and see how it goes. Bella currently rents a one-bedroom apartment in South Carolina and her lease is up in a month, so she might as well.

Bella's recruiter sends her the pay package and she is blown away. She will be making DOUBLE what she is currently making in South Carolina, she is not concerned about finances at all. Her start date is in two weeks, she puts in a two-week notice and starts to prepare for the move.

She buys a new car for the trip because she will need an SUV instead of a car to fit all of her stuff when she drives to Seattle. Her car payment will go from $250 a month to $400 a month but it won't matter because she is making so much more. She also puts the $800 worth of expenses for a cargo carrier and ski equipment (excited for Seattle in the winter) on her credit card (maxing it out) planning on paying it off within the first month after she gets a couple of paychecks. She looks online and finds an amazing place to stay that requires first and last month's rent plus a security deposit upfront (rent is $1,500 per month so it will be $4,500 total). She doesn't have this yet so she puts that on her other credit card. She has about $3,000 in her checking account and figures that will be plenty to pay for gas and food until her first travel check gets deposited.

She leaves for Seattle 10 days before her contract start date. While on the road she has to pay for hotels ($150 a night for 10 nights- $1,500), gas ($300), food ($300) and the sight-seeing she does on the road trip there ($200). She arrives at her new place with $700 in the bank, $4,500 credit card payment, $800 of additional expenses she has yet to pay for, meaning all her credit cards are maxed out. After she arrives she gets a phone call from her recruiter saying that they were unable to get the paperwork processed in time and the facility is pushing her start date back two weeks. Bella starts to panic knowing she only has $700 to live on for the next two weeks and also has to pay her car payment that is due next week. She accepts it and spends the next two weeks relaxing in Seattle but unable to do anything fun since she doesn't have any money.

By the time she starts working she has $100 left in her bank account. Her first day she does computer/charting training. The second day she gets to the floor and realizes this is a cardiac critical care unit for which she has no experience. She will be expected to take care of fresh open-heart patients (of which is most of their patient population), something she has ZERO experience with. This was not communicated with her, is not her fault, but ultimately, the hospital cancels her contract. If she is not trained to care for fresh open hearts, they have no work available for her. She ends up getting paid for two days of work (24 hours) so she doesn't get her full stipends, just her hourly rate since she did not work her 36 hours for the week. That amounts to $336 after taxes, not even enough to make her car payment. She also (after arguing with the recruiter and travel agency) is able to get her $500 travel reimbursement to cover the cost of her traveling to Seattle.

She manages to get lucky and find another job nearby, however, she has to wait two more weeks to start and now has an hour commute each way since she signed a 3-month lease. Everything seems great. She loves her new job and ends up extending spending a year and a half at the same hospital as a traveler. She moves on to travel for three more years with no more issues until she gets a notice that she is being audited by the IRS.

The audit ends up finding that since she never maintained a tax home in South Carolina (she just let her lease end and left) she has been an itinerant employee for the last four years and should have been paying taxes on the money she wrongfully received as tax-free housing and meal stipends. She now owes the IRS $10,000 in back taxes and penalties for each year she has been traveling ($40,000). Over the last four years as a traveler, she has only been able to save $10,000 total and has not been contributing to a 401K so, she has nothing setback for retirement. This absolutely breaks her. She quits travel nursing and goes back to her staff job in South Carolina, with no retirement, no savings, and $30,000 in debt to the IRS.

Bella's story is an important reminder not only to be prepared by having money saved but also to be prepared for tax time and in case you ever get audited. We can also learn that while it may seem like you are getting a giant raise, the costs of duplicating expenses, moving often, increased cost of living wherever you may be going, paying for weekend trips and exploring while on contract, paying for visits home and many other expenses, you may not come out as far ahead as planned.

The moral of the story is to have 3-6 months of expenses saved before quitting your permanent job. Realize that while exciting, travel nursing is not the most stable form of income. Don't do anything drastic or increase your bills to match your new income until you see what is coming and going and how much is left over. Your contract can and will be canceled at any time for any reason.

This can be scary but don't let it be discouraging. Travel nursing is rewarding. You simply must be prepared. Being financially prepared is always a good idea, travel nursing or not. You never know what unexpected expenses may pop up. It is important to find a balance between preparing for the unexpected and enjoying the money you worked so hard to earn.

Getting a Recruiter and an Agency

For this topic, we are going to go pretty in-depth. The idea of a recruiter and an agency is probably something that is very new for people who have no experience with travel nursing. Additionally, the quality of your relationship with your recruiter and agency can make or break your travel nursing experience.

For starters, a discussion of what recruiters do and how to perceive them can help. Recruiters are hired by the travel agency to be the face of the agency. They are in essence the middle man between you, the hospital, and everyone else who works for the travel agency. It is important to know that recruiters are often paid on a structure that involves how many nurses they are able to secure contracts for. Typically, the more nurses they get to sign, the more money they get. This is important to keep in mind because you will need to look for a recruiter that values ensuring you have a good experience over making some quick cash.

Depending on the agency, your recruiter may also be the one who builds your pay package. They may be able to adjust where the money is going and usually have some sort of say what percentage of the bill rate goes where within the limits set by their boss. They are, however, unable to increase the bill rate, so they only have a certain amount of money accessible to work with.

That being said, give your recruiters the benefit of the doubt. Most are interested in making you happy so that you continue to sign contracts with them and they continue to make money. Fostering a good relationship built on mutual trust, understanding, and honesty is incredibly important. Recognize that they are trying to do their job, build a relationship with you, and have a lot on their plate and they should do the same for you. While it is true that the recruiter does not get paid unless you do the work and that they work for you, it is often beneficial to treat them as a part of your team.

Recruiters have many different styles and personalities and you have to find the one that is right for you. This may involve interviewing several different recruiters until you find one that you connect with. In order to do this, you need to decide what you want in a recruiter. Some people want a recruiter who just finds them a job and leaves them alone, others like one who checks in frequently and is eager to help. Decide what you want out of the experience then find someone who is willing to give it to you. There are PLENTY of different recruiters to choose from. Don't settle until you feel comfortable.

You may be wondering how to go about this. My recommendation is to first select an agency. It doesn't matter if you love your recruiter if the agency that they work for doesn't have what you need. If location is important for you, you may want to find out what agencies staff the location you are wanting to go to. Also, consider the differences between a small and a large agency. Small agencies are usually going to have fewer jobs to choose from but your relationship with the agency and the recruiter will feel more personal. Some say they like small agencies because they feel more like a person and less like a number. Large agencies are going to have more opportunities but can sometimes have more automated processes and less time to spend on your individual needs. You will also need to consider the benefits that are important to you. Think of things like insurance, 401K, PTO, cancelation policies, housing processes, and value of pay packages. Even if you find a agency that you like right away, explore a couple of different ones to make sure you aren't missing out on something that would add value to your experience.

So, let's say you did some research online, talked to a few friends to get the names of some agencies, and have narrowed your list of possible agencies down to 5 or 6, maybe even less. The next step is to reach out to a recruiter from the agency and set up a phone call with them. I highly recommend this approach rather than entering your number into contact forms. If you enter your number you will get cold calls from recruiters for the rest of eternity. Also, consider making an email address specifically for travel nursing. That way, if you decide to stop traveling, you can simply not check that email account anymore and your personal email won't be spammed by recruiters.

So, this phone call is going to be like an interview. You are interviewing the recruiter and their agency. This is their chance to impress you. You may want to take notes and write down your general impression after the call as the recruiters and which agency they are from tend to blend together after talking to a couple. They will likely ask you why you are interested in travel nursing to get a feel for how serious you are. They will also ask questions about where you are wanting to go and how much money you are wanting to make. They will also likely tell you a little about their agency and go over some information about the benefits that their agency offers. If you have done your research you should already know most of this information but this is your chance to get any questions you have answered.

You may consider bringing up questions that you have about travel nursing in general to ask the recruiter. This serves two purposes. The first is obviously to get your question answered by someone who should know what they are talking about. The second is to get a feel for how helpful and experienced this recruiter is in general. If they don't know the answer to your question are they willing to find out or direct you to someone who does? Also, don't be afraid to ask them about their experience, and get a feel for how willing they are to connect with you on a more personal level if that is something you value.

The recruiter is going to try to get all your information and start building your profile. Don't let them make you feel rushed into this. Typically, I will give them my email address over the phone at the end of our call, let them send the information we discussed and take a couple of days to look it over and compare it to other information from other recruiters/agencies. I am also always upfront during this conversation that I am looking for a new recruiter/agency and am talking to several different ones and will get back to them. Don't bother filling out information and building profiles with agencies you are not interested in. That just wastes everyone's time.

After you feel comfortable with how many recruiters and agencies you have spoken to, compare them all and pick out your top 2-3. It is considerate to go ahead and reply to the emails from the ones you didn't select and let them know you have chosen to go with a different agency at this time but will keep them in mind for the future. This can be as easy as a generic email copy and pasted to each one and will hopefully keep them from continually reaching out to you when you aren't interested. The top 2-3 that you selected will be the ones you will work with to find your first contract. I am open with those few recruiters that I am working with other agencies to maximize my opportunities. They are generally understanding of this, if not you may reconsider working with them.

Depending on your timeline and how close you are to your planned start date these recruiters may want to start to get your profile ready so they can submit you in a timely manner when a job opens up. Feel free to go through that process with the top 2-3 that you chose.

Build Your Profile

Once you have settled on which agencies you want to work with, you will want to begin to put together your profile with those agencies. Your profile is what the recruiter uses to find you jobs and then submit you to those jobs. Having the profile built ensures that when the job becomes available, the recruiter is able to submit you quickly. Quick submissions increase your chance of landing a job.

To build your profile you will likely need an updated resume and you will need to fill out paperwork which usually includes an agency-specific application and a skills checklist. The process will vary from agency to agency and can get repetitive and time-consuming. Don't get discouraged. It is important to take the time to build profiles with a couple of agencies to help land the perfect job.

While on the topic of profiles and paperwork let's discuss all paperwork that you should go ahead and gather at this time so you will have it available. I recommend making a binder where you keep all this information easily accessible since you will need it every time you sign a contract with a new agency. See the list for items that you should have handy to provide to your agency.

Information for Your Agency

- UPDATED RESUME

- 7-YEAR JOB HISTORY (WITH START AND END DATES) IF NOT INCLUDED ON RESUME

- VACCINATION HISTORY (DON'T FORGET TB AND FLU)

- BLS/ACLS/PALS CERTIFICATIONS AND EXPIRATION DATES

- ANY SPECIALTY SPECIFIC CERTIFICATIONS (FOR EXAMPLE, NIHSS)

- ALL STATE NURSING LICENSES (NUMBER AND EXPIRATION DATE)

- WRITTEN REFERENCES AND CONTACT INFORMATION FOR A MANAGER AND A CHARGE NURSE

- BANK INFORMATION TO SET UP DIRECT DEPOSIT

\# TTTNursing

Get Your License

The timing of this step will be dependent on the many things discussed in the previous section regarding licensing. First, decide where you want to travel. Then figure out how much time you will need to get the appropriate license. We will break this section up into categories depending on your compact status.

If you are a resident in a state that is a compact state and you are planning on traveling to a compact state:

You got it easy! Visit the Board of Nursing (BON) website for your home state and complete the application for a multistate licensure. Once you have this, you will be able to practice in all other compact states. For more information visit https://www.ncsbn.org/compacts.htm

If you are a resident in a state that is a compact state and you are planning on traveling to a non-compact state:

You will need to apply for a license by endorsement in the non-compact state you want to practice in. Visit the BON website for the state you plan on traveling to for more information. The process is different for each state and fees and wait times depend on the individual state. Plan ahead for this as some states can take as long as 3 months, sometimes even longer.

If you are a resident in a state that is a non-compact state and you are planning on traveling to a compact OR non-compact state:

You will need to apply for a license by endorsement in each state you want to practice in. Whether or not the state you want to practice in is compact does not matter because the state you are a resident in is non-compact. Visit the BON website for the state you plan on traveling to for more information. The process is different for each state and fees and wait times depend on the individual state. Plan ahead for this as some states can take as long as 3 months, sometimes even longer.

Plan for Your Permanent Job

Being smart about your current permanent job can make the stress of taking the leap of starting travel nursing less overwhelming. You want to leave on good terms, keep the relationships you have worked to build, and possibly be able to return to work PRN if needed.

First, bare minimum, figure out what the required notice is at your job if you want to quit. Do they need a two-week notice or should you give them a heads up a month before you plan on leaving? The least you can do is adhere to their desired notice time. You may think you never want to come back, but at some point, you may NEED to. Leave on good terms.

You may also consider asking your manager about PRN positions. Some people are able to fulfill the PRN requirements at their permanent job so they are able to work when they come back home between assignments. If the requirement at the hospital is 2 shifts a month, still ask, they may be willing to be flexible in order to have the extra help when you are able to work. For example, if you are going to be gone for 3 months, they may be willing to let you make up your required hours when you return (the 6 shifts you should have worked over the last 3 months).

Also, consider that you will need references for travel assignments. Ask your manager and a charge nurse to write written recommendations for you so you are able to provide them to your travel agency. Continue doing this for every hospital you work at.

Talk to Co-Workers You Trust

Once you are serious enough to put in a notice, start to talk to your co-workers. You may even be able to do this a little before putting in a notice depending on the nature of the relationship with your co-workers (obviously refrain from telling them if they will tell others before you are ready to put in your notice). However, this is an important step because they understand the most about what you are about to do.

Your friends and family are great to talk to but co-workers can be especially helpful. Ask them if there is anything they have noticed that you can work to improve on last minute before you leave. Let them give you a pep-talk about how great of a nurse you are and how you can handle this. Friends and family have probably told you this many times but co-workers are easier to believe because they have actually seen you in action. Let them know that you are wanting to be pushed out of your shell while still comfortable. For example, if you are typically the go-to recorder in codes let them know that you would like a chance at pushing meds so it is fresh when you are in a new environment.

If you have any travel nurses currently working on your unit at your permanent job, even better. Pick their brains. Nurses love sharing their knowledge. Ask them questions and you may even ask if they would be willing to look over your first contract before you sign and give you some insight. Ask them to share the biggest mistake they have made as a traveler so you can avoid it. Ask them what their favorite assignment has been and why. If there are no travelers at your permanent job, you may be able to discuss things with some in online communities.

Leaving your work family can be tough but, they are sure to flood you with confidence and well wishes as you depart. Keep the relationships alive as you travel. Networking is underrated in nursing but can prove to be so important in the future. If nothing else, after a bad shift at a new hospital a call to an old co-worker back home to catch up on what you have missed since you have been gone can be a good stress reliever.

Submit to a Job

The next step is to work with your recruiter to make a timeline for looking at jobs and submitting to open positions. Typically, you see openings start popping up about 4-6 weeks out from your start date. This timeline can vary depending on the time of the year and the location. Just remember, travel nursing jobs tend to be last minute. If they had time to hire permanent staff, they would.

So, the first step of the submission process is to find an available job that you are interested in. Some prefer to give their recruiter a list of criteria and see what the recruiter is able to find. Others like working with agencies that provide a job board to nurses so the nurses can see the available jobs. Either way, make sure your recruiter knows not to submit you to any job without your permission. There are a couple of reasons for this.

First, if you are submitted to the same job by two different agencies sometimes your submissions will be disregarded completely. Second, there are a couple of things that you will want to do before being submitted.

Before being submitted you are going to want to think about the location and the pay package. Start by doing some research on the location. At this point, you may not know the name of the hospital (you can always ask) but do some research for the city provided. See if this is somewhere you would consider going. Then go ahead and look at housing options nearby. See if the location has housing available that fits your needs and analyze the cost of that housing compared to the pay package being offered.

If this initial research does not check out, don't bother submitting to the opening. If you like what you are seeing, give your recruiter the go-ahead to submit you. Feel free to submit to a couple of different positions at the same time. The most important thing is to always make sure before you submit that the information that is available at this point, location and pay, is acceptable to you. If you submit to a job and end up not accepting that job due to the pay package that you knew about before submitting it becomes frustrating to everyone. However, agreeing to submission is not agreeing to accepting the job if offered. If something comes up that you don't like in the interview or you find a position that suits you better, backing out after submission is acceptable.

Before submission, your recruiter will typically ask the best time for a manager at the hospital to contact you for an interview and if you need specifics in your contract regarding schedule (time off during contract, blocked shifts, etc.) so have this information ready!

Interview

The next step after submitting is waiting for an interview! Typically, the nurse manager at the hospital will call you for an interview. They will usually pick one day to call all the applicants and make their decision on who to hire. So, try your hardest to be available when you get that phone call. If you don't answer, they will likely go on to the next applicant and may fill the position before you have a chance to return the call.

The interview will be different depending on the hospital. Some will ask standard interview questions others will focus more on answering your questions. Either way, this will likely be the only time you talk to someone from the hospital before you arrive there if offered the job. Be sure to get all your questions answered in this conversation. See the list for an idea of what to ask during this conversation.

It is important not to verbally accept the position on the phone at this time. If offered the position, a good reply is "I appreciate the offer, I will discuss with my recruiter who will be in contact with you". This way you are not put on the spot and you are able to analyze the information gathered and other options that you have before deciding. Also, it is best to allow the recruiter to draft a formal contract and accept that way as there are agreements between you and your agency that must be decided on before you accept as well.

Information to Ask During the Interview

- CONTACT INFORMATION FOR NURSE MANAGER

- HOSPITAL SIZE AND PATIENT POPULATION:

  - NUMBER OF BEDS (HOSPITAL AND UNIT)

  - LEVEL TRAUMA CENTER

  - PARKING

- WORK ENVIRONMENT:

  - PATIENT RATIOS

  - NURSING ASSISTANTS

  - FLOATING

  - SCHEDULING

  - UNIFORMS

  - CHARTING SYSTEM

#TTTNursing

Accept an Offer

If the interview went well, the hospital will reach out to your agency and offer you the position! This is your last chance to decline the offer. Make sure this is the job you want before signing the contract. After you tell your recruiter that you accept the offer they will draft a contract for you to sign.

It is important to note that this contract is between you and the agency, NOT you and the hospital. Thus, this contract is saying that you agree to work at this place, for this amount of time, for a certain amount of money. The hospital will usually approve the contract but it is not guaranteed that they will follow it. So, if you put certain days off and scheduling requirements in your contract, understand that the hospital should honor it but it is not guaranteed. However, having it in your contract should assure that if you are to break the contract because the hospital will not give you the days off that you put in your contract, there will be no penalties between you and your agency. The hospital likely has a contract with the agency that covers all travelers that the agency sends there.

Do not take signing your contract lightly. Read every single word and don't sign until you understand it. You make want to make special note of a couple of things. First, look at what your contract says about floating. Sometimes hospitals will float travelers first, sometimes you will be required to float to different nearby hospitals within a system. Is there anything in your contract that prevents this?

Second, look at your call off/on-call/canceled shifts requirements. Sometimes hospitals are well staffed because they have too many travelers. If they are overstaffed some will call off travelers first. Is there anything in your contract to prevent you from getting called off once or twice a week with no pay? Along these same lines, realize the difference between "guaranteed hours" and "guaranteed pay". Are they guaranteeing you will be offered your contracted hours every week (whenever they want to offer them, for example, calling you off your scheduled day Wednesday and telling you to work your day off, Saturday, to make up for it) or are they guaranteeing you pay (for example, you get called off Wednesday, and still get paid your normal weekly amount even though you worked fewer hours)?

Third, take a look at the missed shifts policy. When you don't work, the agency doesn't make money. They count on a certain amount of profit from your contract. Your missing shifts means their profit decreases. To make up for this some agencies will penalize you monetarily for calling in or being out sick. What does your contract say about that?

Next, see if there is anything in your contract regarding stipends. If you don't get your contracted hours for the week (for calling in or for being called off) what happens to your stipend? Some agencies will prorate the stipend by the hour (if you aren't working they aren't getting paid and they don't want to pay you), other agencies will guarantee you the stipend since you still have to pay for a place to stay and food to eat.

Additionally, you may want to look at your overtime rate. Remember that when you work overtime, the hospital is paying the agency time and a half of the BILL RATE, not your hourly rate. On this same note, any overtime that you work is extra money for the agency that they didn't plan on making. For this reason, if your hourly rate is $20/hour and your stipends are $30/hour, you want your overtime rate to be AT LEAST $50/hour, hopefully, more. Otherwise, when you are working overtime, you will be making less than what you make for straight time and the agency will be making double or maybe even closer to triple.

Finally, make sure any reimbursements that were agreed upon are outlined in your contract. For example, if a $500 travel reimbursement was presented in the pay package, it should be in the contract with the details of when and how it will be paid out.

Go through this checklist when you get the draft of your contract to make sure everything you need is included in your contract.

- ☐ Approved time off
- ☐ Scheduling agreements
- ☐ Floating
- ☐ Call off/on-call/canceled shifts
- ☐ Missed shifts
- ☐ Stipends for working less than contracted hours
- ☐ Overtime rate
- ☐ Reimbursements

Complete Onboarding

After you sign the contract, you will next work with the agency to complete onboarding. Onboarding will entail gathering all the needed documentation and fulfilling the requirements made by the hospital to work there. For this step, your agency will likely send you to get a physical completed, drug test, and any vaccines that you don't already have. Your agency should pay for all of this.

You will also work with someone to make sure that all information is collected like your licenses and they will verify employment history. This is when that binder of all your information that you made during the profile building phase will come in handy. Make sure to make completing onboarding a priority as not getting onboarding completed in a timely manner can lead to your start date being pushed back.

At this time, your agency may inform you that there are online training modules that need to be done before starting at the facility. It is okay to go ahead and do them before you get there but you should push to be paid for the time that you spend on them. Some facilities have a lot of training modules and they can take a good amount of time to complete. Additionally, it may be wise to wait to complete them until closer to your start date just in case something was to go wrong and your contract ends up getting canceled before you start.

Secure Housing

Once you have a signed contract and completed the onboarding process you can go ahead and secure housing! Most people will have started the housing search process even before submission to an assignment but, now is the time to make a deposit or sign a lease. Depending on what kind of housing you are securing, be cautious with making large deposits to people you have never met for housing you have never seen. It may be smart to put a smaller "holding deposit" down on a place and sign the actual lease once you arrive and see the property.

Do not panic if you don't have housing lined up. Many agencies are able to help with housing searches if you need them to. Also, you can always get a hotel room for a few nights and look for housing once you arrive. It is also worth noting that it may be in your best interest to put preference on places that allow month to month arrangements and don't require the contract commitment. If your contract were to get canceled, it would be nice if you only had to pay the housing until the end of the month rather than the duration of the contract that no longer exists. If a month to month agreement is not possible or it is a significant extra fee, it is always a possibility that you may be able to find another contract within commuting distance if your initial contract gets canceled early.

Pack and GO!

The FINAL step is to pack up your suitcases and get on the road! Most people like to drive to their assignment so that they have a car when they are there. Depending on where you are going, flying may be an option. If you are planning on flying it is possible to get a rental car when you arrive or use public transportation/bike/walk. The biggest piece of advice for this step is not to over pack! You will be surprised at how little you actually need. Just remember that everything you pack you will have to unpack and organize once you get there and pack right back up once your contract ends. The less stuff you bring the easier the whole process is.

If you are staying at a furnished place be in contact with the owner to know what is provided and what you will need to bring. If you have the room you may want to bring basic spices/food staples, cleaning products, toiletries, medicine cabinet essentials, and basic office supplies. If you don't have the room you can always buy that once you get there however it can get expensive to keep buying all the basics every time you move. Be smart and utilize the dollar store and thrift shops to fill in the gaps if you forget something or don't have room.

Make sure you keep receipts from hotels, gas, and food from the trip to your contract. You may need to turn them in for reimbursement of your travel allowance. Also, spend some time planning your route to your destination. Depending on how much time you have you may want to make some scenic stops along the way. You may also want to arrive anywhere from a week to a couple of days before your start date so you can get situated before you have to start working. It isn't uncommon to not get first day instructions until the Friday before your Monday start date. Once you get first day instructions, you may want to do a test run to check out the hospital, parking, and find where you are supposed to go before your first day. Don't forget to factor in unpredictable traffic to your commute. Don't be late on your first day!

You have worked hard for this, you made it. It's time to prove that you have what it takes. Let the small stuff go, enjoy the little things and take in every single new opportunity this adventure has to offer. 13 weeks goes by fast. Whether you are counting down the days till you can leave or slowly soaking up the good that every day brings. Enjoy the moments but don't forget to keep in mind your plan for what is next. Things are always moving as a travel nurse. I know you have what it takes to keep up.

BONUS CONTENT

Here is a bonus section before I send you on your way out into world to spread your wings and fly as a well-prepared travel nurse! This section is going to be a list of tips, FAQ answers, and story time hodgepodges of things I have picked up along the way, laughed at and learned from travelers I have met. Use this section to avoid their mistakes, learn from their fails, and get all your silly questions answered without having to ask for yourself.

1. Use a translator. This is a general nursing tip but especially applicable if you are used to a certain patient population and travel somewhere with a different patient population. A coworker was once trying to explain to a Spanish speaking woman that we needed to get blood from her child. The nurse confused the Spanish word for blood,

"sangre" with "sangria" and the mother left AMA with her child thinking we were trying to give it alcohol.

2. You will likely be drug tested before every new assignment. A coworker once panicked after drug realizing she ate A BUNCH of poppy seed muffins the night before. Her drug test ended up coming back clean after they did some extra testing but I wouldn't risk it.

3. Know what you are signing up for when you hear the words "critical access hospital". It can be a good learning experience if you are used to big facilities but things are often done much differently at these places and resources are limited.

4. Research housing in an area before you submit to an assignment there. Don't be surprised if you

struggle to find places for less than $2,000/month in areas of California, Boston, Seattle, DC, Florida and New York.

5. Account for traffic in bigger cities when choosing places to live before you arrive. 15 miles may not look far on a map but when factoring in traffic you may be signing up for a longer commute than you anticipated.

6. Don't drive to Alaska in September and think you will be able to drive home December!

7. Sometimes facilities will dump the worst patient assignments on the travelers. Don't take it personally. Take it as a compliment. They do it because they know you can handle it and laugh at them all the way to the bank.

8. Don't listen to recruiters when they try to offer you low pay citing that it is because it is your first assignment. Travel assignments don't pay based on experience. Don't settle for a low paying assignment "to get your foot in the door". Find a new recruiter.

9. If you want to go to Hawaii and have pets don't forget to read about rules regarding quarantine for rabies.

10. If you are confused by something, reach out for help. It is the age of the internet. There are tons of travel nurses online that would be happy to mentor you and help answer your questions. No question is a stupid question!

11. Don't assume that because you discussed something with the nurse manager at the hospital in the interview that they will remember it or

honor it. If you need specific scheduling requests, floating policies, or dates off make sure those requests are spelled out in black and white in your contract.

12. Try not to focus too much on being homesick your first assignment. Give yourself time to adjust. Make it your goal to at least finish what you started. 13 weeks goes by fast.

13. Some facilities have specific colors or other uniform requirements. Try to get your scrubs second hand and don't forget to ask in the interview what their requirements are so you can bring that color of scrubs from home if you already have them!

14. If you are taking a local travel assignment (near your permanent residence) there is no such thing as a "50-mile rule". Some recruiters will tell you

that the hospital you are taking the assignment at has to be 50 miles from your permanent residence in order for you to be eligible to receive tax-free housing and meal stipends. This is not true. It should be far enough away that it is reasonable for you not to return home each night and you must be duplicating expenses. This can mean different things depending on the circumstances. If your commute is 30 miles in the snow in Alaska, returning home each night would not be reasonable and you will need a place to stay closer to the hospital. In this case, you should be able to receive tax-free stipends to pay for that place.

15. If you extend your contract at a hospital ask for an extension bonus or a raise. Since you are staying, the hospital does not have to pay to orient a new traveler and the agency does not have onboarding expenses (the time and money they spend on finding you an assignment, paying for physicals

and drug tests, etc.). I also usually suggest a negotiation on your overtime rate as well since agencies are usually making a lot of profit when travelers work overtime and will likely have room to give you a little more of it.

16. Download a free scanner app on your phone. This will make sharing documents with agencies and keeping track of all your paperwork for onboarding a breeze!

17. When looking at 401Ks offered by travel companies keep in mind how long it takes before you are fully vested.

18. The online modules that you have to do for each facility are painfully time consuming. Keep track and see if you are able to print off a report of them from the facility. Sometimes they can be used as CEUs or you may get super lucky and have a

facility that will accept records of completion from another hospital if they use the same or similar training modules.

19. Keep a copy of your all your contracts with your tax information. If you are audited you will need your contract to prove you were employed.

20. Last and final piece of advice! When in Rome, do as the Romans do. Every hospital has a different culture and a different way of doing things. Follow the policies for wherever you are and don't try to change what they are doing (obviously as long as patient safety is not jeopardized). You are there to fill in a gap, provide great care to the patients, and then go on your way. Their drama, their problems, and their processes are not yours to worry about. Keep "the better way to do things" to yourself unless asked and even then, proceed with caution. Have a friendly, non-critical

attitude, do you job, get your pay check, learn from your experience and then carry on with your life.

Made in United States
North Haven, CT
09 November 2021

10981516R00066